800 INDIVIDUAL STATEMENT QUESTIONS
FOR THE MRCPsych PART I

**Dedicated to
Meghna – Our baby girl**

800 INDIVIDUAL STATEMENT QUESTIONS FOR THE MRCPsych PART I

By

Maju Mathews DPM MRCPSYCH
Specialist Registrar
Royal London & St Barts Higher Specialist
Training Scheme
Basildon Hospital
Essex

Provided as a service to medicine by Wyeth Pharmaceuticals

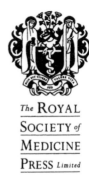

The ROYAL
SOCIETY *of*
MEDICINE
PRESS *Limited*

British Library Cataloguing in Publication Data
A catalogue record for this book is available from the British Library

ISBN: 1 85315 505 5

Typeset by Phoenix Photosetting, Chatham, Kent

Printed in Great Britain by Bell and Bain Ltd, Glasgow

Contents

PREFACE

The MRCPsych is the most important hurdle a psychiatric trainee in the UK faces. This book has been written with the aim of assisting candidates to prepare for the part 1 of this very important exam.

This book has been written in the new format of individual statement questions, which will be the pattern of the exam from autumn 2001. The breakdown of questions from the different subjects reflects that of the actual exam. Further information can be obtained from the college website at www.rcpsych.ac.uk.

This book is structured in the form of four question papers of 200 questions each, with answers and explanations. This is intended to serve two purposes - a systematic way to survey the curriculum of the exam and, as an important way to test one's knowledge, so that gaps can be identified and an attempt made to fill them by further preparation.

I am grateful to those who assessed the questions and helped in the preparation of this book, especially Drs David Tullett, Andrew Black, Hellme Najim, Arghya Sarkhel, J V Patil, B Carr, Vinu George & Manu Mathews.

I am also grateful to everyone at the Royal Society of Medicine press, especially Mr Peter Richardson for their help and assistance in bringing out this book.

I am also grateful to my wife Joanne for her patience and support while I was busy writing.

M.M
August 2001

Paper 1
Questions

Paper I
Questions

1. In visual perception, the same region of the visual cortex carries out localisation and recognition.

2. Figure ground organisation may be reversible.

3. In Gestalt psychology, the determinants of grouping are proximity, closure and similarity.

4. While scanning a picture, the eyes move in a smooth, continuous motion.

5. In multiple personality disorder, the primary personality is usually aware of the existence of the other identities.

6. Most stage 3 and 4 sleep occurs in the first half of the night.

7. According to Winnicott, dreams are a disguised attempt at wish fulfilment.

8. In memory, the left side of the brain is activated during encoding and the right side during retrieval.

9. Short-term memory has a duration of only seconds.

10. In amnesia, semantic memory is lost, but episodic memory is intact.

11. The prototype is a better indicator of a concept than its core properties.

12. All languages have the same set of phonemes.

13. Motivation, in most cases, is as a result of primary re-inforcers.

14. Lesions of the lateral hypothalamus cause lack of hunger.

15. The most common cause of low sex desire is lack of testosterone.

16. Homosexual men can be made heterosexual by being given testosterone.

17. According to the James-Lange theory of emotion, autonomic arousal specific to an emotion mediates the subjective experience of the emotion.

18. Learning is enhanced for mood congruent events.

19. In children, watching television programmes with a violent content has been shown to increase aggression.

20. Alfred Binet devised the earliest intelligence tests.

21. In projective tests, a person has to respond to ambiguous stimuli.

22. People whose spouses are similar to them in personality report greater marital conflict and less satisfaction.

23. People are generally consistent in their behaviours across different situations.

24. People find uncontrollable events to be more stressful than controllable ones.

25. The theory of learned helplessness explains why abused women remain in abusive relationships.

26. People tend to remember reliable and truthful information irrespective of whether it is vivid and shocking.

27. Stereotypes tend to disappear when disconfirming evidence is presented.

28. People do not commit the fundamental attribution error while evaluating their own behaviour.

29. According to Festinger's cognitive dissonance theory, people strive to harmonise their cognitions by removing any inconsistency between them.

30. People who live physically close together are more likely to be friends than those who live far apart.

Paper I
Questions

31. A child shows separation anxiety only on separation from the parents.

32. The use of a transitional object, such as a bear, by a child indicates insecurity.

33. According to Ainsworth, there are three phases to separation from the mother – protest, despair and detachment.

34. Children with early oppositional and deviant behaviour are at no more risk than other children of developing serious problems later on.

35. Fears of the dark and imaginary characters are present in infancy.

36. According to Piaget, assimilation is the modification of cognitive organisation to deal with the requirements of external events.

37. The ability to perform mental operations is a feature of children in the concrete operational stage.

38. Blind babies smile at a later age than babies with normal sight do.

39. According to Erikson, intimacy versus isolation is the dominant theme in adolescence.

40. According to behavioural models of learning, bad behaviours are the causes of mental disorders.

41. In Pavlovian (classical) conditioning, salivation by a dog in response to food is an example of an unconditioned response.

42. Flooding and systematic desensitisation are based on the classical conditioning model of learning.

43. Once an organism engages in certain behaviour, it is usually repeated irrespective of consequences.

Paper I
Questions

44. Variable ratio schedule of reinforcement is more effective in maintaining behaviour than fixed ratio reinforcement.

45. Discriminative stimulus is a stimulus that discriminates between classical and operant conditioning.

46. The generally accepted therapeutic serum lithium level is 0.6 to 1.0 mmol/litre.

47. Constipation is a common side-effect of Fluoxetine.

48. Tricyclic antidepressants can cause a shortening of S-T interval on the ECG.

49. Priapism is a known side-effect of Trazodone.

50. Acute dystonic reaction is more likely to occur with Haloperidol than Chlorpromazine.

51. Dantrolene is a calcium antagonist.

52. The rabbit syndrome caused by neuroleptics is usually present during sleep.

53. Clozapine primarily acts on D4 receptors in the brain.

54. Elevated prolactin while on neuroleptics is mediated by alpha-1 adrenergic receptors.

55. Most drugs taken orally are absorbed into the blood circulation primarily from the stomach.

56. Antagonists and agonists can interact competitively at the same receptor.

57. Water-soluble drugs pass easily across the blood–brain barrier.

58. Clonidine is an alpha-2 agonist.

59. Plasma prolactin level is a marker of central dopaminergic activity.

Paper I
Questions

60. Clozapine induced seizures are best treated with Carbamazepine.

61. Olanzapine is more effective than Risperidone in treating mood symptoms.

62. Clozapine can be given safely during pregnancy.

63. SSRIs can cause akathisia.

64. Monoamine oxidase-A (MAO-A) metabolises dopamine.

65. Pethidine is contraindicated for concurrent use with MAOIs.

66. The presence of psychosis in depression predicts a poor response to ECT.

67. Smoking can lower the levels of tricyclic antidepressants.

68. Lithium is not metabolised in the body.

69. The most important predictor of a good response to treatment with lithium is a family history of bipolar illness.

70. Paranoid features in mania indicate a poor response to lithium.

71. Lithium given in divided doses is less nephrotoxic than when given as a single dose during the day.

72. Aspirin and Diclofenac can be used safely with lithium.

73. Valproate can be given safely during pregnancy.

74. Lamotrigine acts by neuronal membrane stabilisation and inhibiting glutamate release.

75. People with a passive and dependent personality are more likely to develop dependence to benzodiazepines.

76. Binding to D1 receptors correlates with the antipsychotic potency of neuroleptics.

77. Zolpidem acts at the benzodiazepine receptor.

78. The efficacy of a drug is proportional to its potency.

79. Zopiclone does not cause a dependence syndrome.

80. Testing the validity of maladaptive assumptions is an important strategy in psychodynamic therapy.

81. Above average intelligence is an important factor in selecting a patient for psychodynamic therapy.

82. Reduction of anxiety is seen in psychodynamic terms as a secondary gain.

83. Dreaming is an example of primary process thinking.

84. Bion gave the concept of the 'container' and the 'contained'.

85. Transference is absent in healthy individuals.

86. Repression is the pushing away of unacceptable ideas and emotions into the unconscious.

87. Classification in psychiatry is based on symptomatology.

88. Structured interviews like the Present State Examination (PSE) are unsuitable for routine clinical practice.

89. Organic Mental Disorders is not a diagnostic term in the DSM-IV.

90. Mental retardation is classed under Axis II in the DSM-IV.

91. The ICD-10 has a version for daily clinical use and another for research.

92. The most important task of an initial psychiatric interview is to establish a diagnosis.

93. During a psychiatric interview, patients must not be asked about suicide as it may initiate the idea.

Paper I
Questions

94. Compliance with treatment is better if the patient knows the doctor well.

95. In negativism, the patient has negative views of the future.

96. Loosening of associations is pathognomonic of schizophrenia.

97. In stupor, there is an inability to initiate speech or movement.

98. To diagnose schizophrenia according to the ICD-10, the illness must have an onset before the age of 45.

99. The prevalence of schizophrenia differs between countries.

100. Auditory hallucinations are the most common symptom in schizophrenia.

101. Following a psychotic episode, about 25% of patients suffer from depression.

102. Religious delusions are more common in western societies as compared to developing countries.

103. According to Bleuler, hallucinations and delusions are the primary symptoms of schizophrenia.

104. According to the DSM-IV, continuous signs of disturbance must be present for 6 months to diagnose schizophrenia.

105. Schizophreniform psychosis is a term used to describe a psychotic episode which has lasted less than one month.

106. If both the parents are schizophrenic, the children have a 40% risk of developing the illness.

107. Enlargement of the lateral ventricles in the brain is a consistent finding reported in people with schizophrenia.

108. Among people with schizophrenia, about 20% of patients in the acute phase and 10% in the chronic phase commit suicide.

109. In schizophrenia, prominent affective symptoms and a sudden onset predict a good prognosis.

110. Pathological jealousy is more common in females.

111. According to the ICD-10, one episode of mania is sufficient to make a diagnosis of bipolar affective disorder.

112. Relatives of patients with bipolar affective disorder have a greater genetic predisposition to develop mood disorders than relatives of patients with unipolar depression.

113. In bipolar affective disorder, with increasing number of episodes of the illness, the periods of remission between illness become shorter.

114. In bipolar disorder, lithium is more effective in preventing relapse of mania than of depression.

115. Simple phobias generally begin in adolescence.

116. Marital problems are more common among people with agoraphobia than other people of a similar background.

117. In obsessional rituals, there is increased anxiety associated with the failure of the patient to perform the ritual.

118. Conversion symptoms are produced deliberately by the patient.

119. The presence of a physical injury decreases the chances of a person developing Post Traumatic Stress Disorder (PTSD).

120. Post disaster debriefing has been proven to be effective in preventing the later development of PTSD.

121. Sadness with depression occurs in the first stage of normal grief reaction.

122. The rates of suicide increased at the times of the World Wars.

Paper I
Questions

123. Suicide rates increase in pregnancy.

124. A non-dangerous method of self-harm predicts a low risk of subsequent suicide.

125. Puerperal depression is present following 10–15% of all deliveries.

126. In anorexia nervosa, amenorrhoea precedes weight loss in most patients.

127. Growth hormone levels are reduced in anorexia nervosa.

128. Depressive symptoms are more common in anorexia nervosa as compared to bulimia nervosa.

129. Briquet's syndrome was first described by Briquet, a French physician.

130. A normal EEG in a person with convulsions suggests psychogenic convulsions.

131. The absence of withdrawal symptoms on cessation of alcohol use rules out a diagnosis of alcohol dependence.

132. Idiosyncratic alcohol intoxication occurs after the consumption of large amounts of alcohol.

133. Subcortical dementia is characterised by slowing of cognition, and difficulty with complex intellectual tasks.

134. In amnestic syndrome, confabulation is a feature of bilateral hippocampal lesions.

135. Incontinence is a feature of a frontal lobe lesion.

136. In Huntington's disease, insight is lost early on in the course of the illness.

137. Crimes are committed very rarely during epileptic automatisms.

138. Most people with dementia live in residential and nursing homes.

139. Neurofibrillary tangles (NFT) may be seen in the normal elderly brain.

140. Atrial fibrillation is more strongly associated with vascular dementia than Alzheimer's disease.

141. There is a rapid deterioration of the personality in late onset schizophrenia.

142. Retardation or agitation are common presenting features of depression in the elderly.

143. The prevalence of schizophrenia is raised in people with learning disabilities.

144. The greatest advantage of using Methadone in people with opiate dependence is that it is non-addictive.

145. Delirium is the most common psychiatric manifestation in patients with Parkinson's disease.

146. Tics occur at an equal rate in males and females.

147. The content of night terrors is not usually recalled in the morning.

148. Eccentricities of communication, behaviour, and thought are features of schizoid personality disorder.

149. To diagnose depressive disorder, features of depression should have been present for at least 2 weeks.

150. Narcolepsy is associated with sleep paralysis.

151. Patients with depression may show decreased REM latency.

152. Nocturnal penile tumescence is the most useful test to differentiate organically caused impotence from functional impotence.

Paper I
Questions

153. People with anankastic personality disorder can be inflexible and indecisive.

154. Depression is a feature of chronic fatigue syndrome.

155. People who are blind from birth have an increased prevalence of psychiatric disorders.

156. Over half of patients with pancreatic cancer develop depressive symptoms before the appearance of physical symptoms.

157. Depression is the most common psychiatric manifestation of hypothyroidism.

158. The single most common reason among women for admission to medical wards in the UK is deliberate self harm.

159. Withdrawal symptoms on stopping opiates are life threatening.

160. Solvent use is typically a solitary activity.

161. Descriptive psychopathology attempts to explain different psychological symptoms.

162. Delusions as seen in delirium are similar to the delusions of schizophrenia.

163. Behaviour during automatism is usually inappropriate and purposeless.

164. Attention and concentration are impaired in depression.

165. Confabulation is not the same as lying.

166. The body clock runs a little faster than a normal 24-hour cycle.

167. Day dreaming is an example of fantasy thinking.

168. True perception and fantasy always occur separately.

169. In functional hallucination, a percept is needed to produce a hallucination.

170. Hallucinations do not occur when other normal sensory stimuli are received.

171. Autoscopy is the inability to see oneself in the mirror.

172. Olfactory hallucinations with epilepsy strongly suggest the presence of a brain tumour.

173. Extracampine hallucinations are hallucinations in one sensory modality following a stimulus in another.

174. Illusions are a feature of Capgras syndrome.

175. The form of a true delusion can be differentiated from a normal belief.

176. Primary delusions are by definition not understandable to others.

177. Delusional perception is a first rank symptom of schizophrenia.

178. People almost always act on their delusions.

179. Delusions of infidelity are usually resistant to treatment.

180. Primary grandiose delusions may occur in schizophrenia.

181. Nihilistic delusions are a depressive form of self-blame.

182. An obsession is an overvalued idea.

183. Delusional perception can occur in normal people without mental illness.

184. In lateral thinking, the determining tendency of the thought process is sustained.

Paper I
Questions

185. People with flight of ideas may be mute.

186. Crowding of thought is a disturbance of the flow of thinking.

187. Verbigeration is an incoherent mixture of words and phrases.

188. Most patients with schizophrenia demonstrate over-inclusive thinking.

189. The Present State Examination (PSE) uses first rank symptoms as a basis to diagnose schizophrenia.

190. The right side of the brain is the dominant side in most left-handed people.

191. Speech is fluent in receptive dysphasia.

192. In pure word dumbness, writing is preserved, but speech cannot be produced at will.

193. Lesion in the Broaca's area produces expressive dysphasia.

194. Depersonalisation is a subjective experience of an unreal change in the external world.

195. Schizophrenia is the most common diagnosis in people who experience symptoms of depersonalisation.

196. Gastro-intestinal symptoms are the most common symptoms seen in hypochondriasis.

197. Alexithymia is the inability to verbalise emotions.

198. In phobias, fear is in proportion to the demands of the situation.

199. Obsessional thoughts may be delusional.

200. Fugue states generally have a sudden onset.

Paper 1
Answers

Paper I
Answers

1. False

2. True.

3. True.

4. False. Scanning involves successive fixations of the eyes and they tend to be places that are the most informative about the picture.

5. False. The primary identity is unaware of the existence of the other personalities.

6. True.

7. False. This was Freud's theory.

8. True.

9. True. The concept of memory as used in psychiatry is different from that used in psychology. This is the definition used in psychology.

10. False. Semantic memory is intact and episodic memory is lost.

11. False. The core is a better indicator of a concept.

12. False. Every language has a different set of phonemes.

13. False. Secondary reinforcers.

14. True.

15. False. Marital conflicts in people attending sex therapy.

16. False. Sex desire may increase but only towards the same sex.

17. True.

18. True.

Paper I
Answers

19. True.

20. True. Binet was a French psychologist.

21. True. As the stimulus is ambiguous, it is assumed that the individual projects his personality onto the stimulus.

22. False. Less conflict, greater closeness and friendship.

23. False. Behaviour is specific to the situation.

24. True.

25. True.

26. False. People tend to remember vivid information more than non-vivid even if non-vivid is more reliable and informative.

27. False. They tend to persist.

28. False.

29. True.

30. True.

31. False. Attachment figure may be anyone.

32. False. This is a normal phase in development.

33. False. Bowlby stated this.

34. False. They are more prone to problematic behaviours in adulthood.

35. False. Pre-school. Fears in infancy are of pain, loud noise, falling, sudden movements etc.

36. False. This is accommodation.

37. True. 7–11 years. The child recognises the concept of reversibility of mental operations.

Paper I
Answers

38. False. Same age.

39. False. Identity vs confusion. Intimacy vs isolation is seen in early adulthood.

40. False. Learning of maladaptive behaviours, result in mental illness.

41. True. As no learning is involved.

42. True.

43. False. Only if it is reinforced.

44. True. Number of responses keeps varying and the operator cannot predict when the response will occur. (E.g. gambling, slot machines.)

45. False. Discriminative stimulus is a signal that means that reinforcement is available if the operant is made.

46. True.

47. False.

48. False. Prolong S-T interval. Can also cause heart block.

49. True.

50. True.

51. True.

52. False. Disappears during sleep.

53. True.

54. False. D2 blockade.

55. False. Small intestine.

56. True.

Paper 1
Answers

57. False. Lipid soluble drugs pass across the blood–brain barrier.

58. True.

59. True.

60. False. Both can cause blood dyscrasias. Valproate preferred.

61. True.

62. False. Contraindicated.

63. True.

64. False. MAO-A metabolises noradrenaline and serotonin.

65. True.

66. False. Psychosis and biological features predict good response.

67. True. Increases metabolism.

68. True. It is an element and is excreted unchanged.

69. False. Though this is a predictor of a good response, the most important predictor is compliance with treatment.

70. True.

71. False. Once daily dose is safer. The serum trough of lithium levels with once daily dosing allows regeneration and repair of any damaged cells in the kidney.

72. False. Aspirin, Paracetamol & Sulindac are safe. Indomethacin, Diclofenac, Ibuprofen & Piroxicam raise Li levels.

73. False. Teratogenic.

74. True.

Paper I
Answers

75. True.

76. False. Potency of antipsychotic action correlates more closely with D2 receptor binding.

77. True.

78. False. Both are independent of each other.

79. False. Dependence syndrome has been described.

80. False. This is employed in cognitive behavioural therapy.

81. False. Average intelligence is sufficient.

82. False. Example of primary gain.

83. True. In primary process thinking, laws of time and space and distinction between opposites do not apply.

84. True.

85. False.

86. True.

87. True.

88. True. They are inflexible and long.

89. True.

90. True. And personality disorders are also classed under axis II.

91. True.

92. False. Establish rapport and build treatment alliance.

93. False.

94. True. Importance of good therapeutic relationship.

95. False. Patient does opposite of what is asked and resists efforts to make him do what is asked. Seen in schizophrenia.

96. False. Also seen in mania and organic disorders.

97. True.

98. False. No age limit, though usually onset is before 45.

99. False. Generally similar in different countries.

100. True.

101. True.

102. False.

103. False. Primary symptoms are loosening of associations, incongruity of affect and autism.

104. True.

105. False. More than one month but less than six months. Less than one month is brief psychotic disorder.

106. True.

107. True. Anterior and lateral horns. Brains are also lighter and smaller. Reduction in volume of medial temporal structures more on left side of the brain.

108. False. 10% in acute phase and 4% in chronic phase.

109. True.

110. False. Males.

111. False. Two episodes of mood disorder. One episode of mania is bipolar according to DSM-IV.

112. True. Increased risk of both bipolar and unipolar. Unipolar depression breeds true.

Paper I
Answers

113. True.

114. False. Equal.

115. False. Childhood. Social phobia has onset in adolescence. Agoraphobia in early adulthood.

116. False. Patients are from more stable families.

117. True.

118. False. Symptoms produced unconsciously.

119. False. Increases the risk.

120. False. Not been shown to be beneficial. May make symptoms worse.

121. False. Stages: denial, anger, bargaining, depression and acceptance.

122. False. Fell during times of wars and other major disasters.

123. False. Lower.

124. False. Not necessarily.

125. True.

126. False. In about a fifth.

127. False. Increased. Also raised plasma cortisol, and decreased gonadotrophins and T3.

128. False. Depressive symptoms are commoner in Bulimia.

129. False. First described by group of psychiatrists at St Louis.

130. False.

Paper I
Answers

131. False. ICD-10 criteria for dependence: any 3 of a) strong desire to take the substance b) difficulty in controlling intake c) physiological withdrawal d) neglect of alternative pursuits e) use despite harmful consequences f) tolerance.

132. False. Occurs with small amounts. Pathological drunkenness.

133. True. No impairment of language, calculation or learning. Caused by Huntington's, Parkinson's, AIDS, progressive supranuclear palsy etc.

134. False. Occurs with unilateral lesions.

135. True. Personality change, disinhibition, errors of judgement, euphoria, and overfamiliarity.

136. False. Preserved till late.

137. True.

138. False. 80% live in the community.

139. True. In dementia, they are more numerous and have a widespread distribution.

140. False. More closely related to Alzheimer's.

141. False. Personality and affective response are preserved.

142. True.

143. True. Three times increased.

144. False. It is addictive. Form of controlled addiction leading to reduced crime and less chaotic lifestyle.

145. False. Depression.

146. False. More in males and children.

147. True.

Paper I
Answers

148. False. Schizotypal personality disorder.

149. True.

150. True.

151. True.

152. True.

153. True. Obsessional, rigid, upset by change.

154. True. May respond to antidepressants.

155. False. No excess psychiatric problems if blind from birth. If onset is later, it can result in distress.

156. True.

157. True.

158. True. In men it is the second most common reason, next to ischaemic heart disease.

159. False. They cause a lot of discomfort, but are rarely life-threatening.

160. False. It is predominantly a group activity. Only about 5% use is solitary.

161. False. Only describes.

162. False. Delusions are generally fragmented in delirium wheras they are more systematised and complex in schizophrenia.

163. False. It is purposeful and appropriate. Stereotyped activity and repetitive movements may be seen. Awareness of the environment is impaired.

164. True.

165. True. Falsification of memory in a clear consciousness.

166. False. Slower, about 25 hours.

167. True.

168. False. Both are usually admixed.

169. True. But the hallucination is not a transformation of that perception. E.g. hearing voices when the tap is running.

170. False. Can occur.

171. False. This is negative autoscopy. Autoscopy is the experience of seeing oneself and knowing that it is oneself. Also called phantom mirror image.

172. False. May occur with brain tumours, but classically associated with temporal lobe epilepsy.

173. False. Hallucinations experienced outside the limits of the sensory field.

174. False. Capgras syndrome is delusional misidentification.

175. False.

176. True. Secondary delusions usually arise from the underlying mood state and are hence understandable.

177. True.

178. False.

179. True. Very difficult to treat.

180. True.

181. True.

182. False. Overvalued ideas and delusions are not experienced by the subject as senseless, but an obsession is.

Paper I
Answers

183. False. This is a first rank symptom and is hence highly suggestive of schizophrenia.

184. True.

185. True. In severe flight of ideas.

186. False. Seen in schizophrenia. Thoughts are passively concentrated and compressed in the head.

187. False. This is word salad. Verbigeration is the meaningless repetition of specific words or phrases.

188. False. Only about half.

189. True.

190. False. Among left handed poeple, in 60% it is the left side that is dominant. In 20% right and 20% bilateral.

191. True. Difficulty in understanding.

192. True. Can understand speech and writing.

193. True. Lesion in Wernicke's area causes receptive dysphasia.

194. False. This is derealisation.

195. False. Most common is depression.

196. False. Musculoskeletal.

197. True.

198. False. Fear is out of proportion to the demands of the situation.

199. False.

200. True.

Paper 2
Questions

Paper 2
Questions

1. According to Gestalt psychology, people tend to perceive objects as a whole.

2. Perceptual grouping in Gestalt psychology applies only to visual perception.

3. The effects that context has on perception of objects or people are explained by top down processing.

4. Lack of visual stimulation in the first few years of life can permanently impair the visual system.

5. New-borns spend the majority of their sleep time in stage 3 and 4 sleep.

6. People woken up from REM sleep more commonly report dreams.

7. The hippocampus in the brain mediates long term memory.

8. The capacity of short-term memory is 9+2 items.

9. Rehearsing is an effective way of transferring items from short term to long term memory.

10. In memory tests, subjects perform better on recall than recognition.

11. Motor and perceptual skills are lost in amnesia.

12. The English language has about 40 speech sounds.

13. Pleasure is generally associated with stimuli that increases the chances of our or our offspring's survivability.

14. Overweight people tend to eat more in situations of low anxiety as compared to normal weight subjects, who eat more in situations of high anxiety.

15. Women are more concerned about emotional infidelity than sexual infidelity in their partners.

16. The Schachter-Singer theory of emotion states that facial expression determines the subjective experience of the emotion.

17. According to Freud, aggression is induced when expression of instincts is frustrated.

18. Children who are punished severely by their parents are more likely to be aggressive than other children are.

19. In the Stanford-Binet intelligence test, each test item is age graded.

20. The Minnesota Multiphasic Personality Inventory (MMPI) is useful in distinguishing between various forms of psychopathology.

21. Ill-tempered children are more likely to become ill tempered adults.

22. Carl Rogers was the founder of client-centred therapy.

23. According to Maslow's hierarchy of needs, the needs at one level must be satisfied at least partially before those at the next level become important.

24. Humans show more arousal and distress when awaiting predictable shocks.

25. Employed mothers are more likely to develop coronary heart disease than unemployed mothers are.

26. Stress is easier to tolerate when others share the cause of stress.

27. The first impression that one gets about a person has the greatest impact on the overall impression.

28. Fundamental attribution error is the inference that dis-positional (internal) rather than situational attributes are the mediators of behaviour.

Paper 2
Questions

29. Familiarity in general increases interpersonal liking.

30. Individuals exhibit more restraint against indulging in impulsive behaviour than crowds.

31. In Milgram's obedience experiments, the more directly a person knew the victim, the more likely they were to obey the experimenter.

32. Attachment behaviour occurs only to biological parents.

33. Attachment formation begins around 6 months of age.

34. According to Bowlby, the stage of protest is harmless, but despair and detachment can have long term consequences.

35. Parents of aggressive children are often not consistent in their parenting and do not set limits on the child's behaviour.

36. Sexual fears and fears of failure and personal inadequacy are the predominant fears in childhood.

37. Piaget's theory postulates that cognitive development and intelligence develop in a qualitative manner.

38. The ability to think in terms of many possible eventualities is a feature of Piaget's formal operational stage of development.

39. In most western societies, the taboos against feminine behaviour for boys are stronger than masculine behaviour by girls.

40. Erikson's stage of trust vs mistrust corresponds to Freud's oral stage.

41. In Pavlovian conditioning, salivation by a dog in response to a light is a conditioned stimulus.

42. Temporal contiguity between the conditioned stimulus and unconditioned stimulus is the critical factor in the development of classical conditioning.

43. Long term potentiation is the same as long term memory.

44. Operant conditioning increases the likelihood of a response by following the behaviour with a reinforcer.

45. Behavioural assessment does not include explanations of the stimuli presumed to increase or decrease the incidence of the behaviour in question.

46. Serum lithium levels are best measured 24 hours after the last dose.

47. Tricyclic antidepressants can facilitate intraventricular conduction.

48. Hypotension is a common side-effect of Venlafaxine.

49. Lorazepam has a half-life of about 100 hours.

50. Pinpoint pupils are a feature of heroin withdrawal syndrome.

51. Nefazodone acts primarily on serotonin 1A receptors.

52. Postural hypotension is mediated primarily by alpha-1 adrenergic receptors.

53. The presence of metabolising enzymes in the liver does not affect the rate of drug absorption into the circulation.

54. An antagonist drug always produces the opposite effect to an agonist.

55. First order kinetics state that the change in concentration is independent of the concentration of the drug.

56. D2 receptor occupancy rates of more than 90% are required for most antipsychotics to exert their effects.

57. Phase 1 drug trials refers to a drug being administered to animals.

Paper 2
Questions

58. The presence of dopamine increases prolactin levels.

59. Antipsychotics decrease the turnover of brain dopamine.

60. Olanzapine causes a lesser increase in prolactin levels than Risperidone.

61. Tardive dyskinesia is commoner in females.

62. Among tricyclics, tertiary amines are more potent at blocking 5HT uptake.

63. Antiepileptics can increase tricyclic levels.

64. Monoamine oxidase inhibitors are the drugs of choice in atypical depression.

65. Monoamine oxidase-A (MAO-A) is the predominant form of MAO in platelets.

66. Beta-1 receptor upregulation is a postulated mechanism of action of tricyclic antidepressants.

67. A washout period of 2 weeks is necessary while switching from Fluoxetine to a MAOI.

68. Lithium is excreted unchanged by the kidney.

69. Mania followed by depression has a better response to lithium than depression followed by mania.

70. Lithium is present in breast milk.

71. Valproate has a similar efficacy to lithium in mania.

72. Carbamazepine can increase warfarin levels.

73. Zopiclone has a half-life of about 1 to 3 hours.

74. Dopamine D4 receptors are functionally similar to D2 receptors.

75. A benzodiazepine with a short half-life is more likely to cause dependence than one with a longer half-life.

76. The effects of Zopiclone can be reversed with Flumazenil.

77. According to Freud, castration anxiety is the predominant fear of 2-year-olds.

78. Motivation only for symptom relief is a necessary criterion for brief dynamic therapy.

79. The main psychodynamic defence mechanism in paranoid personality disorder is projection.

80. According to Melanie Klein, the depressive position predisposes to depression in later life.

81. Some degree of idealisation is normal part of an analytic relationship.

82. Transference occurs only in the analytical setting.

83. Carl Jung gave the concept of Animus and Anima.

84. The ICD-10 attempts to explain the aetiology of different psychiatric disorders.

85. In psychiatric interviewing, it is preferable to obtain a history from a relative before making a formulation.

86. ICD-10 is a multiaxial system of classification.

87. The DSM-IV has a broader definition of schizophrenia than the ICD-10.

88. Diagnoses of personality disorders have greater interclinician reliability than organic and psychotic disorders.

89. In a psychiatric interview, it is important to take into account the patient's view of the aetiology of his illness.

90. A patient who cries during an interview should be allowed to cry.

Paper 2
Questions

91. Mannerisms are repetitive purposeless movements.

92. Mood and affect are defined differently.

93. The prevalence of schizophrenia is equal in men and women.

94. People with schizophrenia are classically described as having difficulty interpreting proverbs.

95. Social withdrawal is the most commonly seen feature in chronic schizophrenia.

96. In schizophrenia, paranoid symptoms are more common in middle age than in young adults.

97. Auditory hallucinations and delusions are first rank symptoms of schizophrenia.

98. DSM-IV criteria for diagnosis of schizophrenia is based on Schneider's first rank symptoms.

99. Relatives of people with schizoaffective disorder are at increased risk of schizophrenia but not mood disorders.

100. Crow described the concept of Type I and II schizophrenia.

101. The risk of bipolar disorder is increased in first degree relatives of schizophrenics.

102. Obstetric complications at the time of birth result in an increased risk of schizophrenia.

103. Patients with schizophrenia living with their families generally have a lower rate of relapse than those living in hostels.

104. De Clérambault syndrome is commoner in women than men.

105. Rapid cycling bipolar disorder is commoner in males than females.

106. The mean age of onset of bipolar disorder is 28 years.

107. The density of brain 5HT2 receptors is decreased in patients dying by suicide.

108. The earlier the age of onset of depression, the greater the risk of recurrence.

109. Early morning awakening is a feature of generalised anxiety disorder.

110. Avoidance and anticipatory anxiety are characteristic features of phobic disorder.

111. The prevalence of obsessive compulsive disorder is equal in males and females.

112. Dissociative disorders have a mean age of onset of 50 years.

113. People who suffer from PTSD have increased rates of deliberate self-harm and substance abuse.

114. In patients who suffer from terminal illnesses, emotional reactions are more common in the young as compared to the elderly.

115. Abnormal grief is more likely when the death is sudden and unexpected.

116. Suicide rates are highest in the winter.

117. People who indulge in deliberate self-harm rarely commit suicide.

118. In people with gender identity disorder, cross-dressing begins before the age of four.

119. Puerperal psychosis generally has an onset within two days of delivery.

120. Maternity blues are best treated with antidepressants.

Paper 2
Questions

121. Anorexia nervosa generally begins between the ages of 12 and 14 years.

122. Males with anorexia nervosa have a better prognosis than females.

123. In bulimia nervosa, patients have a loss of control over eating.

124. Somatisation in females is associated with alcoholism in male relatives.

125. Men are more sensitive to the harm inducing effects of alcohol.

126. Gilles de la Tourette syndrome is commonly seen in early adulthood.

127. Disorientation for time is a feature of amnestic syndrome.

128. Lesions of the dominant parietal lobe cause visuo-spatial problems.

129. Pick's disease affects women more often than men.

130. Post stroke depression is more common following a left-sided stroke.

131. Early onset Alzheimer's disease is associated with the E4 allele of apolipoprotein E.

132. Lewy body dementia can present with psychotic symptoms and fluctuating consciousness.

133. Mania in the elderly more often presents with irritability and agitation than elation of mood.

134. Senile plaques and neurofibrillary tangles may be present in Lewy body dementia.

135. Onset of depression after the age of 70 predicts a good prognosis.

136. About 50% of people with learning disabilities suffer from epilepsy.

137. In alcoholic hallucinosis, the hallucinations are usually tactile.

138. In narcolepsy, the sleep attacks are characteristically non-refreshing.

139. Premature ejaculation is usually caused by organic factors.

140. Withdrawal symptoms from methadone begin within one to three days after the last dose.

141. Insomnia is a characteristic feature of seasonal affective disorder.

142. The rate of major depression does not differ across races.

143. Panic disorder has the highest comorbidity with depression.

144. The father is most often the perpetrator in child abuse.

145. Multiple personality is classified under personality disorders.

146. People with schizoid personalities may be successful in occupations requiring solitary work.

147. Depressive disorder should not be diagnosed in a person with borderline personality disorder.

148. Decisions made by groups are more extreme than those made by individuals.

149. Emotional distress can precipitate asthmatic attacks.

150. Psychiatric disorders are more common in pregnant women than non-pregnant women of the same age.

151. People with cancer have increased rates of depressive disorder as compared to people with other physical illness.

Paper 2
Questions

152. The severity of mental disorders with exogenous steroid administration is dependent on the dosage of the steroids.

153. The risk of suicide is lowered among people who call the Samaritans.

154. 60% of alcohol abusers have raised MCV levels.

155. The incidence of schizophrenia is increased among cannabis users.

156. Amphetamine use can result in a psychotic illness indistinguishable from schizophrenia.

157. Flashbacks can occur after months or even years following LSD use.

158. Phenomenology involves the observation and categorisation of abnormal psychic events.

159. In clouding of consciousness, disorientation for time occurs earlier than that for place and person.

160. The presence of perseveration suggests a functional illness.

161. Objective assessment of the duration of time elapsed in depressed patients is accurate when compared to euthymic patients.

162. Completion illusions are removed by attention.

163. A true hallucination occurs spontaneously.

164. Synaesthesia is the experience of hearing colours and seeing sound.

165. Pseudohallucination occurs in inner subjective space.

166. The presence of pseudohallucinations strongly suggests an organic illness.

167. People who experience sensory deprivation may start to hallucinate.

168. A delusion of worthlessness is an example of a primary delusion.

169. Delusional atmosphere may be seen in the prodromal phases of schizophrenia.

170. Persecutory delusions may help in protecting the patient from low self-esteem.

171. Cotard's syndrome is a feature of severe depression in the elderly.

172. In circumstantial thinking, the subject takes a long time to answer questions and goes into unnecessary detail.

173. Speech is usually coherent in severe loosening of associations.

174. Bulbar and pseudobulbar palsy can result in logoclonia.

175. In conduction dysphasia, the patient cannot speak and write, but can repeat whatever is spoken to him.

176. In pure agraphia, speech is normal.

177. Alogia means poverty of thought.

178. The presence of depersonalisation invariably indicates the presence of a mental illness.

179. Hypochondriacal symptoms are left sided in the majority of patients.

180. Transsexualism is the wearing of clothes of the opposite sex.

181. Anhedonia means an inability to experience pleasure.

182. Patients recovering from a severe depressive episode are at an increased risk of suicide.

183. Manic patients can be extremely distractible.

Paper 2
Questions

184. Insight is preserved in obsessive compulsive disorder.

185. Fluctuating consciousness is a feature of delirium.

186. Hemisomatognosia is the neglect of one half of the body.

187. Somatopagnosia is an inability to recognise a neurological deficit as occurring to oneself.

188. Beck's depression inventory is a self-rating scale.

189. Depersonalisation usually lasts from minutes to hours.

190. Hypochondriacal symptoms may be held with delusional intensity.

191. A person suffering from OCD realises that the thoughts arise from within him.

192. Performance of compulsive rituals does not result in pleasure.

193. Overvalued ideas are always false.

194. Hamilton depression rating scale (HAM-D) is a self-rating scale.

195. The presence of constant pain without exacerbating or relieving factors suggests pain of psychogenic origin.

196. In somatic passivity, the patient experiences an alien drive to carry out a motor activity.

197. Personal construct theory can be investigated using behavioural analysis.

198. The ability of thinking to flow towards its goal is called the determining tendency.

199. All delusions are paranoid in phenomenological terms.

200. Delusions may be alterable by persuasion.

Paper 2
Answers

Paper 2
Answers

1. True.

2. False. Also auditory.

3. True. When context is appropriate, it facilitates perception, when inappropriate, it impairs perception.

4. True. Greatest vulnerability is in the first two years though the critical period may last as long as eight years.

5. False. They spend about half of their time in REM sleep.

6. True.

7. True. The frontal cortex mediates short-term memory.

8. False. 7 plus or minus 2 items.

9. True.

10. False. Recognition is better than recall.

11. False. They are retained.

12. True. All languages have limited speech sounds, but rules for combining them make it possible to produce thousands of words.

13. True.

14. False. Overweight people eat more in situations of high anxiety and in response to external cues.

15. True. Men are more worried about sexual infidelity.

16. False. The emotional experience depends on the physiological arousal and the cognitive appraisal of the situation.

17. True.

18. True.

Paper 2
Answers

19. True.

20. False. This is used to assess personality.

21. True. Generally, but not always.

22. True. Based on the principle that every individual has the motivation and ability to change and he or she is the best person to decide on the direction of change.

23. True.

24. False. Predictable shocks induce less arousal and distress and they are perceived as less aversive than unpredictable shocks.

25. True. Employed women are not at increased risk. The likelihood of disease increases with the number of children for working mothers, but not for homemakers.

26. True.

27. True. Primacy effect.

28. True.

29. True.

30. True. There is loss of identity (deindividuation) in a crowd, hence less restraint.

31. False. The less contact one has with a victim, the more likely one is to obey the experimenter.

32. False.

33. True.

34. False. Protest and despair are harmless. Detachment begins a few weeks after separation and increases with subsequent separations.

Paper 2
Answers

35. True.

36. True.

37. True.

38. True.

39. True.

40. True.

41. False. This is a conditioned response. The light is the stimulus.

42. False. The predictive relation, i.e. there must be a higher probability that an unconditioned stimulus will occur when a conditioned stimulus has been presented than when it is not.

43. False. This is the process of a neuronal synapse becoming more efficient and firing readily following a learning episode.

44. True.

45. True. The described assessment is called a functional analysis. Behavioural analysis involves a record of the behaviour, its incidence, duration and intensity.

46. False. 12 hours.

47. False. Inhibit conduction.

48. False. Hypertension is more common.

49. False. 7 to 35 hours. Diazepam about 100 hours.

50. False. Opiate use. Withdrawal causes dilated pupils.

51. False. 5HT 2A receptors.

52. True.

53. True. The liver is exposed to the drug only after absorption.

54. False. Not necessarily.

55. False. This is zero order kinetics. In first order kinetics, the rate of absorption depends on the dose remaining to be absorbed.

56. False. Between 65% and 85%.

57. False. This is the time when a drug is given to humans for the first time. This is to establish whether and at what dose the new compound may be safely administered to humans. The drug may be given to healthy volunteers or patients.

58. False. Dopamine in the tubuloinfundibular system inhibits prolactin release from the pituitary.

59. False. Increase turnover.

60. True.

61. True.

62. True. Secondary amines block noradrenaline uptake.

63. False. Decreases.

64. True.

65. False. MAO-B in platelets. MAO-A is found predominantly in the intestinal mucosa. Both are found in the brain and liver.

66. False. Downregulation.

67. False. Five weeks. Two weeks for other SSRIs.

68. True.

Paper 2
Answers

69. True.

70. True.

71. True.

72. False. Decrease warfarin levels by enzyme induction.

73. False. 3 to 6 hours.

74. True. D2, D3 and D4 receptors are similar. D1 and D5 are similar.

75. True. E.g. Lorazepam is more likely than diazepam to cause dependence.

76. True.

77. False.

78. False.

79. True.

80. False. Is a normal stage.

81. True.

82. False. Can occur in all relationships.

83. True.

84. False. Makes diagnosis based on symptoms.

85. True.

86. False. Single axis. DSM-IV is multiaxial.

87. False. Narrower definition.

88. False. Organic and psychotic disorders have greater inter-clinician reliability.

89. True.

90. True.

91. False. This is stereotypy. Mannerisms are repetitive, voluntary, purposeful movements.

92. True. Mood is a prolonged prevailing state. Affect is used to describe specific feelings directed towards objects.

93. True. Later age of onset in women.

94. True. Exhibit concrete thinking. Proverb interpretation requires abstract thinking.

95. True.

96. True. In the young, the common symptoms are thought disorder, withdrawal, insertion, mood disturbance etc.

97. False. Third person and command hallucinations and delusional perception are first rank symptoms.

98. False. ICD-10 based on Scheidnerian symptoms.

99. False. Risk of both increased.

100. True.

101. False.

102. True.

103. False. Higher, especially in families with high expressed emotion.

104. True. The subject, usually a woman, believes that a person of higher social standing is in love with her.

105. False. More common in females. Responds better to Valproate.

Paper 2
Answers

106. False. 21 years.

107. False. Increased.

108. True.

109. False. Suggests depression.

110. True.

111. True.

112. False. Onset is much earlier. Extremely rare after 40 years.

113. True.

114. True.

115. True.

116. False. Highest in spring.

117. False. Suicide risk in people who harm themselves is raised 100 times in the subsequent year.

118. True.

119. False. Within the first 2 weeks. Rarely in the first 2 days. Maternal blues begin 2 to 4 days post partum.

120. False. They are self-limiting.

121. False. Adolescence, 16 to 17 years.

122. True.

123. True.

124. True. And sociopathy.

125. False. Women.

126. False. Onset in childhood.

127. True.

128. False. This is a feature of non-dominant lobe lesion. Dominant lobe lesion causes dysphasia, apraxia, finger agnosia, agraphia etc.

129. True.

130. True.

131. False. Late onset is associated with E4.

132. True. Also fluctuating consciousness and increased sensitivity to neuroleptics.

133. True.

134. False. Senile plaques are present but no neurofibrillary tangles.

135. False. Good prognostic factors – onset before age 70, short duration of illness, good premorbid adjustment, absence of physical illness, and good recovery from previous episodes.

136. False. One third.

137. False. Auditory.

138. False. The patient wakes up refreshed.

139. False. Psychological factors.

140. True.

141. False. Hypersomnia, hyperphagia.

142. True. Generally same rates among different races.

143. True.

Paper 2
Answers

144. True.

145. False. Classed under dissociative disorders.

146. True.

147. False.

148. True.

149. True.

150. False. Pregnancy protects against psychiatric illnesses and suicide.

151. False. Same rates as other physical illness.

152. False. Not dependent on the dose.

153. False. Increased in the subsequent years.

154. True.

155. True. Risk increased 2.5 times. Six fold increase in heavy users.

156. True.

157. True.

158. True.

159. True.

160. False. Almost always a sign of organic brain disease.

161. True. Because of low mood, people feel that time is passing slowly.

162. True. Occur because of inattention.

163. True.

Paper 2
Answers

Paper 2
Answers

164. True.

165. True.

166. False. Does not suggest any mental illness.

167. True.

168. False. Secondary delusion, because of the mood state.

169. True.

170. True.

171. True.

172. True.

173. False. Incoherent.

174. False. Causes dysarthria.

175. False. Cannot repeat, but can speak and write.

176. True. Agraphia without alexia–normal understanding of written and spoken material.

177. True.

178. False.

179. True. Three fourths.

180. False. This is transvestism. Transsexuals believe that they belong to the opposite gender.

181. True.

182. True. During severe depression there might be anergia and retardation and lack of motivation. On partial recovery, with the regaining of energy and motivation, patients may actually carry out the act.

Paper 2
Answers

183. True.

184. True. Patient realises that his thoughts are senseless.

185. True.

186. True. Usually left side.

187. False. This is anosognosia. Somatopagnosia is an inability to recognise a body part as one's own.

188. True.

189. True. Can last longer.

190. True. Can be a primary or secondary delusion, obsessional idea, overvalued idea or arise as a result of hallucinations.

191. True.

192. True. Only a reduction in anxiety.

193. False. May be true, but dominates the person's life.

194. False. Observer rated.

195. True. Physical pain usually increases and decreases, and is also relieved by various measures.

196. False. This is passivity impulse. Somatic passivity is the belief that outside influences are playing on the body.

197. False. Investigated using repertory grid.

198. True.

199. True. Paranoid means self-referent and all delusions are self-referent.

200. False. One of the criteria of calling a belief a true delusion is that they are not alterable, and held with firm conviction.

Paper 3
Questions

Paper 3
Questions

1. In perception, the difference between bottom up and top down processes are that the former are driven solely by the input, whereas the latter are driven by the person's knowledge and expectations.

2. NREM sleep is characterised by a wide-awake brain in a virtually paralysed body.

3. In REM sleep, stimuli from other parts of the body are blocked from entering the brain and there may be no motor outputs.

4. Visual coding for memory is better in children.

5. When new items are added to short term memory, items encoded earlier are displaced.

6. The more items there are in short-term memory, the faster retrieval becomes.

7. Long term memory representation is mainly visual and acoustic.

8. Recall is best when the dominant emotion during retrieval is the same as that during encoding.

9. Children are born with an ability to identify phonemes in the language of their parents.

10. Reward is mediated through the mesolimbic dopaminergic system.

11. Lesions of the venteromedial hypothalamus cause increased appetite.

12. Food deprivation leads to subsequent anorexia nervosa.

13. Reminiscence therapy is useful in the treatment of depression.

14. Homosexuals generally experience same sex attraction by the age of 3 years.

15. The higher the level of emotional arousal, the better the performance.

16. Men with extremely high testosterone levels are more likely to have high status positions than low status positions in society.

17. Girls and boys tend to imitate aggressive behaviour with the same frequency.

18. IQ tests are poor at predicting job successes.

19. In MMPI tests, it does not matter whether what the person being tested says is really true.

20. Inter-rater reliability is better for thematic apperception tests than for Rorscharch tests.

21. Freud's structural model of the mind consists of the conscious, preconscious and the unconscious.

22. The superego develops in response to parental rewards and punishments.

23. There are good co-relations between trait measures on personality tests and actual behavioural observations.

24. Pleasurable situations may be stressful.

25. The crucial factor in type A personality predisposing them to disease is not urgency or competitiveness but hostility.

26. All defence mechanisms are pathological.

27. Schemas are helpful in processing information rapidly and efficiently.

28. Strong and consistent attitudes are a better predictor of behaviour than weak and ambivalent attitudes.

29. Physical attractiveness is important over the long-term course of a relationship.

Paper 3
Questions

30. Asch did experiments on conformity.

31. Decisions following discussions by groups are generally well thought-out, rational decisions.

32. Attachment behaviour and stranger anxiety develop at approximately the same age.

33. Clear cut attachment develops in a child by three months of age.

34. The potential damage of separation from the mother can be counterbalanced by good social contact with others.

35. Aggressive behaviour in children generally tends to be consistent over time and situations.

36. About two-thirds of the children could be grouped as easy in the New York longitudinal study.

37. A child can see the world from another person's point of view in Piaget's pre-operational stage.

38. Puberty has an earlier age of onset in boys than in girls.

39. According to Kohlberg, most adults operate at stage 6, i.e. the highest stage of moral reasoning.

40. Boys who mature early are more likely to be emotionally unstable and have poor self-control than those who mature late.

41. In classical conditioning, when a conditioned response has been associated with a particular stimulus, similar stimuli may evoke the same response.

42. In learning, there may be structural changes at the neuronal level.

43. The law of effect promotes survival of the fittest responses.

44. If a behaviour that has been established is reinforced only occasionally, there is rapid extinction.

45. Avoidance responses are very difficult to extinguish.

46. In operant conditioning, a positive reinforcer is an event whose onset increases the probability that a voluntary response will occur again.

47. In exposure and response prevention, the patient watches another person perform the behaviour he is unable to perform himself.

48. High lithium levels may occur with a high sodium diet.

49. Tardive dyskinesia disappears during sleep.

50. Abrupt withdrawal of phenelzine can cause seizures.

51. Buspirone acts mainly on 5HT 1A receptors.

52. Weight gain with psychotrophics is mediated by blockade of noradrenaline uptake.

53. Prenatal exposure to lithium is associated with Ebstein's anomaly.

54. Lipid soluble drugs pass more readily across membranes than water soluble ones.

55. First pass effect is the metabolism of a drug by the liver before it reaches the systemic circulation.

56. Glutamate is an excitatory neurotransmitter.

57. Drugs that block presynaptic dopamine receptors increase dopamine synthesis and release.

58. Clozapine is a dibenzodiazepine.

59. Tardive dyskinesia may be present in schizophrenics untreated with medication.

60. Anticholinergic drugs must be regularly given to patients receiving neuroleptics.

Paper 3
Questions

61. Akathisia affects about 50% of people on neuroleptics.

62. Jaundice with phenothiazines is dose dependent.

63. Amitryptiline is metabolised to nortryptiline.

64. Cimetidine increases tricyclic antidepressant levels.

65. Foods like cheese should be avoided while taking MAOIs as they may cause hypotension.

66. Venlafaxine is a selective noradrenaline reuptake inhibitor.

67. Phenothiazines can raise tricyclic levels.

68. The combination of SSRI and MAOI can be used in cases of severe resistant depression.

69. Patients achieve steady state blood levels about three days after starting lithium.

70. Family history of bipolar disorder indicates a poor response to lithium.

71. Decreased T3 is usually the first sign of hypothyroidism in patients treated with lithium.

72. Valproate is the preferred anticonvulsant in clozapine induced seizures.

73. The GABA-A receptor complex is associated with a chloride channel.

74. Tricyclics generally cause weight loss.

75. Low serum cholesterol is seen in anorexia nervosa.

76. Financial benefits are an example of primary gain.

77. According to Melanie Klein, splitting and projection are seen in the paranoid-schizoid position.

78. According to Winnicott, the primary motivational drive of a person is to seek a relationship with others.

79. Psychodrama is the psychological understanding of famous plays.

80. History that patients give about drugs and alcohol should be taken at face value.

81. Psychiatric diagnoses are categorical rather than dimensional.

82. The use of video and audio feedback is the most effective way of enabling doctors to develop interviewing skills.

83. In waxy flexibility, the patient's limb remains in the position in which it is placed.

84. Visual hallucinations are common in schizophrenia.

85. Persecutory delusions are specific to schizophrenia.

86. Flattening of affect is the diminution of emotional response.

87. The ICD-10 requires that symptoms be present for one month to make a diagnosis of schizophrenia.

88. Catatonic symptoms are rarely seen now in clinical practice.

89. Delusions and hallucinations are elaborate and organised in hebephrenic schizophrenia.

90. Monozygotic twins have a 50% risk of developing schizophrenia.

91. People with schizophrenia have a higher mortality than the general population.

92. Paranoid schizophrenia has a later age of onset than other forms of schizophrenia.

Paper 3
Questions

93. Patients with bipolar disorder have more episodes of illness than patients with unipolar depression.

94. Agoraphobia generally has a good prognosis.

95. Depersonalisation disorder has an onset in early adult life.

96. Young widowers and elderly widows are at highest risk of suicide following bereavement.

97. Absence of grief is pathological.

98. Deliberate self-harm is more prevalent in the lower social classes.

99. ECT is the treatment of choice in postpartum psychosis.

100. Postpartum psychosis is associated with a complicated delivery.

101. Late onset anorexia nervosa has a better prognosis than early onset of the illness.

102. Sensory changes in conversion disorders do not conform to the anatomical neural innervation of the part affected.

103. Munchausen's syndrome is commoner in women than men.

104. Delirium tremens develops within 24 hours of stopping drinking by an alcohol dependent person.

105. One fourth of patients in a surgical ICU suffer from delirium.

106. Men are more commonly affected with Huntington's disease than women.

107. Elderly patients with depression have a higher mortality rate than those without depression.

108. Alzheimer's disease is best diagnosed by a CT scan.

109. The rate of suicide is increased in patients with somatisation disorder.

110. Aggressive and violent behaviour is associated with decreased levels of CSF 5-HIAA levels.

111. Tourette's disorder is associated with OCD.

112. The squeeze technique is used in the treatment of secondary impotence.

113. Panic attacks may be treated with an infusion of sodium lactate.

114. Methylphenidate can cause growth retardation in children.

115. The most important task of a psychiatrist is to give advice.

116. Withdrawal symptoms on stopping heroin typically last two to three weeks.

117. Bipolar disorders can be differentiated from schizophrenia on the basis of response to neuroleptics.

118. In somnambulism, there is amnesia for the episodes.

119. Immediate recall is preserved in amnestic syndrome.

120. The incidence of schizophrenia has doubled in the past 100 years.

121. Reproductive rates in people with schizophrenia have increased in the past few decades.

122. ECT may be given in pregnancy.

123. Risperidone is a benzosoxazole derivative.

124. Transference is a response to countertransference.

125. High premorbid educational achievement is a risk factor for suicide in schizophrenia.

Paper 3
Questions

126. Reciting the months of the year in reverse order is a test for long term memory.

127. Hyperphagia is a feature of bulimia nervosa.

128. Persisting cognitive impairment following head injury is greatest when there is a post-traumatic amnesia of between 6 and 12 hours.

129. Confusion and ataxia are common features of Wernicke's encephalopathy.

130. Cataplexy is a feature of neuroleptic malignant syndrome.

131. Simple phobias are associated with mitral valve prolapse.

132. The prevalence of depression is greater in rural than urban areas.

133. Borderline personality disorder is more commonly diagnosed in women than men.

134. Rapid cycling bipolar disorder requires the presence of at least three affective episodes in twelve months.

135. Cognitive impairment occurs early in the course of Huntington's disease.

136. ICD-10 diagnosis of PTSD requires that symptoms arise within six months of the traumatic event.

137. Prolactin response to infusion of L-tryptophan is increased in depressed patients.

138. Depressive disorders are more common in the higher social classes.

139. Cotard's syndrome is more common in the elderly.

140. People with schizoid personality disorder have a predilection for solitary activities.

141. Cerebellar lesions are seen in Korsakoff's psychosis.

142. Cerebellar atrophy is a feature of Pick's disease.

143. Schneiderian first rank symptoms may be seen in mania.

144. Persecutory delusions are a characteristic feature of paranoid personality disorder.

145. Difficulty in exhaling is a somatic symptom of anxiety.

146. Failure of superego development is suggested as one of the core features of antisocial personality disorder.

147. The prevalence of personality disorders decreases with age.

148. Cognitive behavioural therapy has been shown to be helpful in relieving symptoms of chronic fatigue syndrome.

149. The most common cause of atypical chest pain without an organic cause is depression.

150. People who develop profound deafness at a very young age are more prone to emotional and behavioural disorders than those who develop deafness at a later age.

151. Risk of suicide in cancer is increased in later stages of the disease.

152. Vitamin B12 deficiency can cause dementia.

153. People with depression and panic disorder are at a greater risk of committing suicide than people with depression alone.

154. The rates of deliberate self-harm are rising.

155. The peak age of deliberate self-harm in men is lower than that for women.

156. Opiates are abused for their euphoriant effects.

Paper 3
Questions

157. Patients withdrawing from benzodiazepines may experience withdrawal symptoms for months.

158. Long term cannabis use is associated with lack of motivation and apathy.

159. Death can result from even occasional use of ecstasy.

160. Heightened consciousness can occur with the use of illicit drugs.

161. Clouding of consciousness in delirium characteristically occurs in the afternoon.

162. Violence is rare during automatism.

163. In déjà vu, the person has feelings of familiarity for events experienced for the first time.

164. In jamais vu, an experience that a person has experienced before is not associated with the appropriate feeling of familiarity.

165. Pseudologica fantastica is synonymous with confabulation.

166. Sense perception is experienced as real and to be acted upon.

167. Affect illusions are banished by attention.

168. Visual hallucinations characteristically occur in organic states.

169. Formication is the sensation of insects crawling under the skin.

170. Hallucinations of the bereaved are usually pseudohallucinations.

171. Extracampine hallucinations are hallucinations produced in one modality following a stimulus in another.

Paper 3
Questions

172. Olfactory hallucinations may be seen in anorexia nervosa.

173. Voices in alcoholic hallucinosis respond very well to neuroleptics.

174. Delusional perception is an example of a secondary delusion.

175. Delusions are always self-referent.

176. Delusional memory is also called retrospective delusion.

177. Deafness and social isolation result in maintenance of delusions.

178. The cultural and social background of the patient determines the content of delusions.

179. In de Clérambault's syndrome, a woman believes that a man of higher social standing is in love with her.

180. Koro is seen in Malaysia.

181. In la folie à deux, the person who acquires the delusion first is usually the dominant partner.

182. Delusional perception is a two-stage process.

183. The most common psychiatric symptom seen in multiple sclerosis is euphoria.

184. In flight of ideas, there is a loss of connection between each of the two sequential ideas expressed.

185. Retardation of thinking is a characteristic feature of depression.

186. Thought blocking is a first rank symptom.

187. The inability to give literal meanings to words or sentences is called concrete thinking.

188. Asyndesis is the lack of adequate connection between two consecutive thoughts.

Paper 3
Questions

189. A voice giving a running commentary is a first rank symptom.

190. All passivity experiences are first rank symptoms.

191. Logoclonia may occur in Parkinsonism.

192. Naming and reading are impaired in pure word deafness.

193. Speech is fluent in jargon dysphasia.

194. In alexia with agraphia, the patient is unable to read, write, speak or understand speech.

195. In doppelgänger phenomenon, the patient is aware of oneself being both outside and inside himself.

196. Amok is characterised by depersonalisation, rage, automatism and violent acts.

197. Wearing clothes of the opposite sex does not lead to genital excitement in transsexualism.

198. Diminished dreams and fantasies are a feature of alexithymia.

199. Phobias are not under voluntary control.

200. Catatonia is not abolished by voluntary activities.

Paper 3
Answers

Paper 3
Answers

1. False. The other way round.

2. False. This is REM sleep.

3. True.

4. True.

5. True. To make way for the new items.

6. False. It becomes slower.

7. False. It is based on meanings.

8. True.

9. False. Children can discriminate between different phonemes in any language. Over the first year of life, they learn phonemes relevant to their language and lose the ability to discriminate between other phonemes.

10. True.

11. True.

12. False. Deprivation leads to overeating and subsequent weight gain.

13. False. Used in dementia.

14. True.

15. False. Performance increases with arousal till a level of optimum arousal, then decreases (Yerkes-Dodson curve).

16. False. Men with high testosterone levels are more likely to have low status positions in society.

17. False. Girls are much less likely to imitate aggressive behaviour unless it is specifically reinforced.

18. True.

19. True. This is a criterion-keyed method and hence what is important is the fact that he or she says it.

20. True.

21. False. This is the topographical model. Structural model consists of the id, ego and the superego.

22. True.

23. False.

24. True.

25. True.

26. False. Defence mechanisms are pathological only when they become the dominant mode of responding to problems.

27. True.

28. True.

29. False. This is important in the short term.

30. True.

31. False. In groups, because of a strong desire to maintain group consensus, members spend more time rationalising their decisions, rather than examining them for strengths and weaknesses. This is called groupthink.

32. True. About six months.

33. False. Between seven months and two to three years.

34. True.

35. True.

36. False. About 40% were classed as easy.

Paper 3
Answers

37.   False. Pre-operational stage is characterised by ego-centricity. Thinking is characterised by realism, animism and artificialism. The ages of two to seven years is the pre-operational stage.

38.   False. Girls – 11 years, boys – 13 years.

39.   False. Only 10% function at the stage of highest moral reasoning.

40.   True.

41.   True. This is called generalisation.

42.   True.

43.   True. Stated by Thorndike. The law of effect selects from a set of random responses just those responses that are followed by positive consequences. Seen in operant conditioning.

44.   False. Behaviour can be maintained even if it is reinforced only a fraction of the time–partial reinforcement.

45.   True.

46.   True.

47.   False. This is modelling. In exposure and relapse prevention, the person is exposed to the fear and prevented from engaging in the anxiety relieving compulsion. Used in OCD.

48.   False. Seen with a low sodium diet.

49.   True.

50.   True.

51.   True.

52.   False. Blockade of H1 receptors.

53. True.

54. True.

55. True.

56. True.

57. True.

58. True.

59. True.

60. False. Only if needed.

61. True.

62. False. This is an idiosyncratic reaction.

63. True.

64. True.

65. False. Cause hypertensive crisis. These are tyramine containing foods. MAO normally inactivates tyramine in the gut. When this is inhibited, it results in the release of noradrenaline, hence causing hypertension.

66. False. It is a 5HT and noradrenaline inhibitor.

67. True. They inhibit their metabolism.

68. False. It is absolutely contraindicated.

69. False. Steady state levels in about a week.

70. False. It is a good prognostic factor.

71. False. Raised TSH is one of the earliest signs.

72. True.

Paper 3
Answers

73. True.

74. False. Doesn't cause either hypothyroidism or diabetes insipidus.

75. False. Hypercholesterolaemia.

76. False. Secondary gain.

77. True.

78. True. Object relations theory.

79. False.

80. False.

81. True.

82. True.

83. True.

84. False. Suggest organic disorders.

85. False. Occur in a range of conditions including schizophrenia, mania, depression, substance misuse, organic disorders etc.

86. True.

87. True.

88. True.

89. False. In hebephrenia, affective symptoms and thought disorder are more prominent. Delusions and hallucinations are fragmented and not organised.

90. True.

91. True.

92. True.

93. True.

94. False. Agoraphobia lasting more than one year changes little in the next five years.

95. True.

96. False. Young widows and elderly widowers are at the highest risk of suicide following bereavement.

97. True.

98. True.

99. True.

100. False. No relationship.

101. False. Better prognosis when it begins at a younger age and the duration of illness is short.

102. True. Varies according to the patient's concept of illness.

103. False. More in men.

104. False. Begins within two to three days.

105. True.

106. False. Sex ratio is equal.

107. True.

108. False. Diagnosed clinically. Definite diagnosis is only possible on autopsy.

109. False.

110. True.

Paper 3
Answers

111. True.

112. False. Treatment of premature ejaculation.

113. False. Sodium lactate precipitates panic attacks.

114. True.

115. False.

116. False. Lasts 7–10 days.

117. False. Both respond to neuroleptics.

118. True.

119. True.

120. False. May be decreasing.

121. True.

122. True.

123. True.

124. False. Transference is the feelings and emotions evoked in the patient towards the therapist. Countertransference is the feelings towards the patient evoked in the therapist.

125. True.

126. False. Test of concentration.

127. True.

128. False. Greatest when post traumatic amnesia lasts more than 24 hours.

129. True. These with ophthalmoplegia constitute the classical triad of Wernicke's.

130. False. Rigidity, confusion, hyperpyrexia, autonomic instability along with raised creatinine kinase levels are seen in neuroleptic malignant syndrome.

131. False. Panic disorder is associated with mitral valve prolapse.

132. False. Urban communities have a greater prevalence of depression than rural.

133. True.

134. False. Four or more episodes.

135. False. Later on in the illness.

136. True.

137. False. Prolactin response is decreased in response to L-tryptophan in depressed patients.

138. False. Bipolar disorder is more common in the higher social classes.

139. True.

140. True.

141. True.

142. False. Generalised atrophy in the frontal and temporal lobes is seen. Cerebellum is usually spared.

143. True. About 20–30% of people with mania show first rank symptoms.

144. False. May be seen in many other disorders.

145. False. Difficulty inhaling is seen in anxiety.

146. True.

Paper 3
Answers

147. True.

148. True.

149. False. Panic disorder is the most common of nonorganic atypical chest pain.

150. False. Those who develop deafness later in life are more prone to emotional and behaviour disorders.

151. False. Risk of suicide is increased in the early stages after diagnosis.

152. True.

153. True.

154. True.

155. False. Men have a higher average age for deliberate self-harm than women do.

156. True.

157. True.

158. True. Acute effects are anxiety, paranoia, toxic confusional state etc.

159. True.

160. True. LSD, amphetamines etc.

161. False. It occurs in the evenings.

162. True.

163. True.

164. True.

165. False. Pseudologica fantastica is fluent plausible lying. Confabulation is a falsification of memory in a clear consciousness.

166. True.

167. True.

168. True.

169. True. Seen in cocaine addiction and alcohol withdrawal.

170. True.

171. False. They are hallucinations experienced outside the limits of the sensory field.

172. False.

173. False. Respond to stopping drinking.

174. False. It is a primary delusion.

175. True.

176. True.

177. True.

178. True.

179. True.

180. True.

181. True.

182. True.

183. False. Depression in up to 50%. Euphoria in about 10%.

Paper 3
Answers

184. False. In flight of ideas, the logical connection between two sequential ideas expressed is retained. It is lost in loosening of association.

185. True.

186. False.

187. False. Concrete thinking is giving literal meanings to words or sentences, i.e. inability to think abstractly.

188. True.

189. True.

190. True.

191. True. This is the spastic repetition of syllables.

192. False. Naming and reading are intact. Comprehension and repetition are impaired.

193. True. But there may be such gross disturbance of words and syntax that speech is unintelligible.

194. False. Patient can speak. Understanding is preserved.

195. True.

196. True. Seen in Malaysia.

197. True. Clothes of the opposite sex are worn only for personal gratification.

198. True.

199. True.

200. False. Catatonia is a state of increased tone in muscles at rest. It is abolished by voluntary activity.

Paper 4
Questions

Paper 4
Questions

1. To perceive an object in motion, it is necessary for the image to move across the retina.

2. Stimuli that are not attended to by a person are filtered out completely.

3. Depth perception is present in newborn infants.

4. REM sleep plays an important role in the processing and storage of memories.

5. Chunking of information can increase short-term memory.

6. Information retention lasting from minutes to years occurs in long term memory.

7. Forgetting from long term memory is usually due to decay of the information.

8. In acquiring knowledge of concepts, core concepts are learned through explicit teaching.

9. Damage to the brain structures that mediate long-term memory does not lead to impairment of learning.

10. The rewarding consequences of an action are an indicator of whether an action is worth repeating.

11. Obese individuals are more sensitive to internal hunger cues than external cues.

12. The anatomical development of a female embryo requires the presence of female sex hormones.

13. Childhood gender non-conformity may predict adult homosexuality.

14. The sensations of pleasure change from childhood to adulthood.

15. High testosterone levels are associated with higher levels of aggression.

16. The expression of aggression acts as a cathartic, resulting in the reduction intensity of aggressive feelings and actions.

17. The Wechsler adult intelligence scale (WAIS) is divided into two parts, verbal and memory scale.

18. Rorschach test is an example of a projective test.

19. Children with dependency traits in childhood usually grow up to become aggressive men.

20. According to Carl Rogers, the wider the gulf between the ideal self and the actual self, the more dissatisfied and unhappy a person is.

21. Kelly's personal construct theory is based on personality tests.

22. According to the Holmes & Rahe social readjustment rating scale, divorce is the most stressful event.

23. Seligman's experiments on learned helplessness were done on chimpanzees.

24. Depressed individuals attribute negative events to external causes.

25. People with many social ties are less likely to suffer from stress related illness.

26. In most mixed sex interactions, women appear more knowledgeable than men do.

27. According to Festinger's cognitive dissonance theory, dissonance-causing behaviour may lead to attitude change.

28. Physical attractiveness is not an important factor in interpersonal attraction.

29. Passionate love is important for sustaining long term relationships.

Paper 4
Questions

30. A person who collapses is more likely to be helped by bystanders on a crowded street than on a street with very few people.

31. In a group, the presence of a minority with a different point of view can influence the opinion of the majority.

32. Physical abuse and battering of a child is incompatible with the development of attachment behaviour.

33. Attachment is the same as bonding.

34. Piaget conducted the strange situation experiments with children.

35. Aggression in children is mediated mainly by environmental factors.

36. The opportunity to play with other children is necessary to learn how to express aggression.

37. Fears of unfamiliarity and strangeness are present in the first half of infancy.

38. According to Piaget, object permanence is attained in the sensorimotor stage of development.

39. According to Piaget, the concept of conservation is established in the concrete operational stage of development.

40. Fathers are more concerned than mothers about sex-typed behaviours in children.

41. In classical conditioning, if an association between an unconditioned stimulus and conditioned stimulus is reinforced repeatedly, there is extinction of the response.

42. Habituation is the process when an organism learns to strengthen its reaction to a weak stimulus if a threatening stimulus follows.

43. The more the time difference between the operant response and the reinforcer, the greater the response strength as the organism has been waiting longer for the reinforcer.

44. Punishment is more effective than reward in eliminating unwanted behaviour.

45. An infant has the same visual acuity as an adult by the age of six months.

46. A negative reinforcer is an event whose onset will decrease the probability of a voluntary response.

47. In chaining, complex behaviour is taught by breaking it into smaller parts.

48. Chlorpromazine is less likely than haloperidol to cause orthostatic hypotension.

49. ECT and phenothiazines can precipitate manic episodes in patients with bipolar disorder.

50. Tremor is a known side-effect of diazepam.

51. Seizures are a feature of heroin withdrawal.

52. Most drugs follow first order kinetics.

53. The assessment of the therapeutic value of a new drug is done in Phase II clinical trials.

54. Benzodiazepines act on GABA-B receptors.

55. Dopamine D1 receptors stimulate adenylate cyclase.

56. Tardive dyskinesia disappears on stopping neuroleptics.

57. Acute dystonias are more common in the elderly.

58. Antipsychotics may be reintroduced in the majority of people who have had neuroleptic malignant syndrome.

Paper 4
Questions

59. Tricyclics potentiate the action of warfarin.

60. MAOIs exert their action primarily by inhibition of MAO-B.

61. Mianserin can cause blood dyscrasias.

62. Tricyclics increase stage 4 sleep.

63. SSRIs do not cause extrapyramidal side effects.

64. Lithium has a high affinity for serum albumin.

65. Acamprosate reduces the effect of excitatory amino acids.

66. Depot haloperidol is administered every 2 weeks.

67. Coarse tremors are a side-effect of lithium.

68. Valproate is the drug of choice in rapid cycling bipolar affective disorder.

69. Gabapentin is not protein bound or metabolised in the body.

70. Plasma half-life of drugs is decreased in the elderly.

71. Clozapine binds with high affinity to D4 receptors.

72. Nicotine withdrawal symptoms are more severe in men.

73. Ability to tolerate anxiety without regression is important in brief dynamic therapy.

74. The internalised parent figures of the superego are formed from reality and fantasy.

75. According to Freud, the ages between six and puberty constitute the latency period.

76. The patient disagreeing with the therapist indicates that there is a poor therapeutic relationship.

77. Primary process thinking is the operating system of the unconscious.

78. A person who kicks the wall after arguing with his wife is exhibiting the defence mechanism of acting out.

79. If two disorders respond to the same drug, it means they share the same aetiology.

80. DSM-IV uses operational criteria to make psychiatric diagnoses.

81. Axis III of the DSM-IV refers to psychosocial and environmental problems.

82. A 'colour blind' approach must be taken while assessing patients from ethnic minority populations.

83. Empathy is also called sympathy.

84. It is important to elicit a psychosexual history in the initial interview.

85. The presence of psychomotor retardation is incompatible with mania.

86. Perseveration is commonly associated with schizophrenia.

87. Mutism is the absence of speech in a clear consciousness.

88. The mean age of onset of schizophrenia is five years earlier in men than women.

89. Social withdrawal in schizophrenia is a sign of depression.

90. Post schizophrenic depression may be a response to recovery of insight.

91. Kraepelin proposed the name schizophrenia.

92. Epilepsy in learning disabilities is more common in females.

Paper 4
Questions

93. Temporal lobe epilepsy and amphetamine abuse can result in schizophrenia.

94. Schizotypal disorder is classified along with schizophrenia in the ICD-10.

95. Thought processes are relatively intact in paranoid schizophrenia.

96. Schizoaffective disorder with predominantly manic symptoms has a better prognosis than that with depressive symptoms.

97. MRI studies have shown a reduction in the volume of the temporal lobes in schizophrenia.

98. The prognosis for schizophrenia is better in western societies with advanced psychiatric services than in less developed countries.

99. Folie à deux usually occurs within members of the same family.

100. Rates of bipolar disorder are higher in women than men.

101. Life events are more strongly associated with an earlier age of onset of depression.

102. In mania, antipsychotics produce an earlier symptomatic improvement than lithium.

103. There is an increased prevalence of depression in patients with anxiety disorders.

104. Panic disorder is commoner in women.

105. Behavioural therapy is more effective in controlling obsessional thoughts than compulsive rituals.

106. Complex PTSD is more likely following type I trauma.

107. Children and the elderly are more likely to develop PTSD.

108. Mechanic suggested the concept of sick role.

109. The highest rate of rise in suicides has been among young men.

110. Suicide in people with schizophrenia is more likely among the young, early on in the course of their illness.

111. Family history of multiple sclerosis is a risk factor for suicide in patients with the illness.

112. People with puerperal psychosis are more prone to develop bipolar affective disorder.

113. Bradycardia is seen in anorexia nervosa.

114. Patients with bulimia nervosa are usually of normal weight.

115. Conversion symptoms are more common in developing countries.

116. Cosmetic surgery can be beneficial in body dysmorphic disorder.

117. People of Afro-Caribbean origin in the UK have a higher prevalence of alcohol related disorders.

118. Amnestic syndrome is characterised by a disorder of recent memory.

119. Dominant temporal lobe lesions cause an impairment of intellectual functioning.

120. Grandiosity is the most common psychiatric manifestation of neurosyphilis.

121. The prevalence of psychiatric disorders is raised in people with epilepsy irrespective of how well the epilepsy is controlled.

122. Neurofibrillary tangles are intracellular structures.

Paper 4
Questions

123. The risk of developing a manic episode increases with age.

124. Insight is maintained to a late stage in vascular dementia.

125. Alcoholic hallucinosis occurs in a clear sensorium.

126. Brain tumour is an absolute contraindication to ECT.

127. The rituals in OCD are ego-dystonic.

128. The absence of mental illness is a necessary criterion for a person to stand trial.

129. Withdrawal symptoms from heroin begin within six to eight hours of the last dose.

130. Narcolepsy is associated with hypnagogic hallucinations.

131. Slow wave sleep may be decreased in the elderly.

132. In depression, there is a greater REM frequency in the first half of sleep.

133. Attention seeking behaviour is a feature of OCD.

134. Sex therapy is usually ineffective for lack of desire.

135. Overgeneralising is a feature of graded task assignment in CBT.

136. Inconsistent and impulsive parenting is a contributing factor in development of antisocial personality disorder.

137. Emotionally unstable personality disorder is a classification in the ICD-10 but not DSM-IV.

138. People with borderline personality disorder rarely commit suicide.

139. Schizoaffective disorder has a better prognosis than mood disorders.

140. Insistence on symmetry in OCD is associated with a good prognosis.

141. Dementia is a common complication in people with AIDS.

142. The most common psychiatric disorder in people diagnosed with cancer is depression.

143. In women with breast cancer, psychiatric morbidity is less after conservative treatment with lumpectomy, than following mastectomy.

144. Paranoid symptoms are the most common psychiatric manifestation of Cushing's syndrome.

145. People with symptoms of hopelessness are at increased risk of suicide.

146. Treating people for depression has not been shown to decrease suicide rates.

147. Most patients with deliberate self-harm have a diagnosable psychiatric disorder.

148. Disulfiram acts by blocking oxidation of alcohol.

149. Tolerance for opiates remains at a high level even when the drug is stopped.

150. A dependence syndrome can develop with cannabis use.

151. Craving for cocaine can re-emerge after months of abstinence.

152. Insight is best described as present or absent.

153. Binswangers disease is a type of vascular dementia.

154. Twilight state may be seen in temporal lobe epilepsy.

155. A visual pseudohallucination becomes more clear by looking directly at it.

Paper 4
Questions

156. Patients with confabulation may be highly suggestible.

157. Approximate answers in a clear consciousness are a characteristic feature of Ganser's syndrome.

158. Micropsia means seeing objects as smaller than their real size.

159. Pareidolic illusions are removed by attention.

160. A true hallucination has the full force and impact of a real perception.

161. Clang associations may be seen in flight of ideas.

162. The commonest psychiatric diagnosis associated with autoscopy is delirium.

163. Pseudohallucinations resemble fantasy more than true hallucinations.

164. In reflex hallucinations, a stimulus in one modality produces a hallucination in another.

165. Visual hallucinations are not seen in blind people.

166. The content of a delusion may at times be true.

167. Autochthonous delusions arise suddenly out of the blue.

168. The voices in schizophrenia usually decrease when the patient becomes drowsy.

169. People with delusions make external, stable and global attributions for positive events.

170. Persecutory delusions are characteristic of schizophrenia.

171. The primary phenomenon in Capgras syndrome is a hallucination.

172. Religious delusions are caused by excessive religious beliefs.

Paper 4
Questions

173. Overvalued ideas often dominate the life of the person who holds them.

174. Delusion is a formal thought disorder.

175. The determining tendency of thought is often weakened in flight of ideas.

176. In derailment of thinking, there is a preservation of normal chain of associations with a bringing together of heterogeneous elements.

177. Tangentiality is an example of formal thought disorder.

178. Overinclusive thinking in schizophrenia arises from an inability to preserve conceptual boundaries.

179. Thought withdrawal is a passivity phenomenon.

180. Somatic passivity is similar to haptic hallucination.

181. Aphonia is the loss of ability to vocalise.

182. In nominal dysphasia, the patient is unable to produce names.

183. In primary motor dysphasia, speech is affected but writing is intact.

184. Neologism is the creation of new words and can occur in schizophrenia.

185. Trance and possession disorders may occur in normal healthy people.

186. Windigo is seen in Mexico and North Africa.

187. Transvestism is a disorder of core gender identity.

188. People who engage in exhibitionism also engage in other sexual deviations.

Paper 4
Questions

189. Anxiety in generalised anxiety disorder is confined to specific situations.

190. The mini mental state examination (MMSE) is a useful diagnostic tool for dementia.

191. Echopraxia is the imitation of the examiner's actions by a patient in spite of being asked not to.

192. In phenomenological terms, dysmorphophobia is an over-valued idea.

193. Prosopagnosia is an inability to recognise faces.

194. Pain of psychological origin tends to be well localised.

195. Thought disorder is a negative symptom of schizophrenia.

196. A person suffering from phobia usually realises the senseless and irrational nature of his fears.

197. Memory loss is a characteristic feature of dissociative fugue.

198. The form of different mental illnesses may vary across cultures, but the content is usually the same.

199. In transient global amnesia, the memory loss tends to be selective for certain events.

200. Dexamethasone suppression test may be used to monitor the progress of depressive illness.

Paper 4
Answers

Paper 4
Answers

1. False. Stroboscopic motion e.g. movies where a series of still pictures create the impression of motion.

2. False. There is partial processing of non attended stimuli.

3. False. Begins to appear by three months and is fully established by six months of age.

4. True.

5. True. Chunking is recording material into larger meaningful units using long term memory.

6. True.

7. False. It is usually due to a failure of retrieval.

8. True. Core concepts are learned through explicit teaching while prototypes are acquired through experience.

9. False. It does, as learning makes extensive use of prior knowledge.

10. True.

11. False. Obese people eat in response to external cues e.g. sight of food even if not hungry.

12. False. Development of a female embryo only requires the absence of male hormones.

13. True.

14. False. The sensations of pleasure are the same, but the ideas associated with the sensation and the source of pleasure change.

15. True.

16. False. Aggression tends to breed aggression.

17. False. The two scales are the verbal and performance scales.

18. True.

19. False. Children with dependency traits grow up to become calm, warm, sympathetic individuals and are more likely to have intact marriages.

20. True.

21. False. Based on the cognitive model.

22. False. Death of spouse is perceived as the most stressful event.

23. False. Dogs.

24. False. Depressed individuals attribute negative events to internal causes and vice versa.

25. True. They have lesser feelings of hopelessness and also an increased ability to cope.

26. False. Men appear more knowledgeable than women do as they control situations more and also question and interact more.

27. True.

28. False.

29. False. Though it is essential for the short-term success of a relationship, compassionate love, equality, trust, tolerance, warmth and affection are more important in sustaining long term relationships.

30. False. People are less likely to help when others are present.

31. True.

32. False. Attachment can develop in these circumstances. Intense social interaction is sufficient.

Paper 4
Answers

33. False. Attachment is the relationship between infant and caregiver and takes several years to develop. Bonding is the initial human attachment in the first few days of life.

34. False. Mary Ainsworth.

35. False. Environmental and biological factors.

36. True.

37. False. These are present in the later half of the first year.

38. True.

39. True.

40. True.

41. False. Extinction occurs when the association is not re-inforced.

42. False. This is sensitisation. Habituation is the weakening of a reaction if there are no serious consequences.

43. False. Immediate reinforcement is more effective than delayed.

44. False. The effects of punishment are not predictable and they may elicit more unwanted behaviours.

45. False. Between one and five years.

46. False. This is punishment.

47. True.

48. False. More likely.

49. False. ECT can precipitate mania, not phenothiazines.

50. False.

Paper 4
Answers

51. False.

52. True.

53. True. Phase II trials aim to establish clinical efficacy, incidence of side-effects, define appropriate doses and provide detailed pharmacological and metabolic data.

54. False. They act on GABA-A receptors.

55. True.

56. False. May increase.

57. False. Commoner in young males.

58. True.

59. True.

60. False. MAO-A.

61. True.

62. True. They also reduce the number of awakenings, increase the latency to onset of REM sleep and reduce the duration of REM sleep.

63. False. SSRIs can cause EPSEs. Fluoxetine reduces the turnover of dopamine in the basal ganglia.

64. False. Lithium is not bound to serum proteins and is excreted unchanged by the body.

65. True. Acamprosate decreases the effect of glutamate.

66. False. Given every four weeks.

67. False. Fine tremor is a side effect. Coarse tremor is a sign of toxicity.

68. True.

Paper 4
Answers

69. True.

70. False. Plasma half-life is increased in the elderly.

71. True.

72. False. They are more severe in women.

73. True.

74. True.

75. True.

76. False.

77. True. Uses mechanisms such as displacement, condensation and symbolisation.

78. False. Acting out is expressing unconscious emotional conflicts or feelings directly in action without being consciously aware of their meanings.

79. False.

80. True.

81. False. General medical condition.

82. False.

83. False.

84. False.

85. False. May be present in manic stupor.

86. False. It is associated with organic disorders.

87. True.

88. True.

89. False. May be, but not necessarily. It is a recognised negative symptom of schizophrenia.

90. True.

91. False. Eugen Bleuler.

92. False. Commoner in males.

93. False. They cause schizophrenia like syndrome. The diagnosis of schizophrenia requires that organic factors be ruled out.

94. True.

95. True.

96. True.

97. True.

98. False. Better prognosis in developing countries. Patients in developing countries are more likely to achieve complete remission.

99. True.

100. False. Equal in males and females.

101. False. Life events have a greater association with a later age of onset, when there is relatively less genetic loading.

102. True. Antipsychotics have an effect on psychotic symptoms and overactivity while lithium primarily treats elated mood. However, lithium produces an overall greater improvement than antipsychotics.

103. True.

104. True.

105. False. More effective in controlling compulsive rituals.

Paper 4
Answers

106. False. Type I trauma is a short, unexplained traumatic event, e.g. rape, natural disasters etc. It is more likely to lead to classic re-experiencing and may also show quicker recovery.

Type II trauma is multiple, chronic, repeated traumas, e.g. ongoing physical and sexual abuse. This can cause complex PTSD and has a poorer prognosis.

107. True.

108. False. Suggested by Parsons. Mechanic suggested the concept of illness behaviour.

109. True.

110. True.

111. False.

112. True.

113. True. Also delayed gastric emptying, constipation, hypotension, hypothermia, leucopenia etc.

114. True.

115. True.

116. True.

117. False. Lower than white populations.

118. True. also inability to learn new information and recall previously learned knowledge.

119. True. Can also cause epilepsy, schizophrenia, personality change, emotional instability and aggressive behaviour.

120. False. Dementia and depression are more common.

121. False. The prevalence of psychiatric illnesses is raised in chronic severe epilepsy. However, if the epilepsy is well controlled, there is little increase in the prevalence of psychiatric disorders.

122. True.

123. False. Depressive disorder increases with age, not mania.

124. True.

125. True.

126. False. Caution advised.

127. True.

128. False.

129. True.

130. True.

131. False. Slow wave sleep is usually increased in the elderly.

132. True.

133. False.

134. True.

135. False. One of the cognitive distortions causing depression.

136. True.

137. True.

138. False. People with borderline personality disorders have an increased rate of death by suicide as compared to the general population.

Paper 4
Answers

139. False. Better than schizophrenia but worse than mood disorders.

140. False. Poor prognosis.

141. False. Minor cognitive impairment is more common.

142. False. Adjustment disorder is the most common diagnosis.

143. False.

144. False. Depression.

145. True.

146. False. Does reduce suicide rates.

147. False. Most people with deliberate self-harm have some affective symptoms but very few have a full psychiatric disorder. However in completed suicides the vast majority have a psychiatric disorder.

148. True.

149. False. Tolerance diminishes very rapidly on stopping opiates.

150. True.

151. True. Craving can re-emerge on exposure to psychological and social cues.

152. False.

153. True. Arteriosclerotic disorder affecting subcortical areas.

154. True. Characterised by an abrupt onset and end, variable duration of few hours to weeks and occurrence of un-expected violent acts or emotional outbursts.

155. False. Removed by attention.

156. True.

157. False. Clouding of consciousness is a feature. Other features are disorientation, somatic conversion symptoms and pseudohallucinations.

158. True. Occur in parietal lobe lesions, epilepsy etc.

159. False.

160. True.

161. True.

162. False. Depression is more commonly associated with autoscopy.

163. False. Pseudohallucinations resemble true hallucinations more than fantasy.

164. True.

165. False. May be seen.

166. True. It is the evidence presented for holding the belief that is important.

167. True.

168. False. May increase.

169. False. People with delusions make external attributions for negative events and internal attributions for positive events.

170. False. Also occur in depression, mania, organic disorders etc.

171. False. This is a delusional misidentification.

172. False.

Paper 4
Answers

173. True.

174. False.

175. True.

176. False. This is fusion. In derailment, there is a breakdown in associations and there is interpolation of thought bearing no understandable connection with the chain of thoughts.

177. True.

178. True.

179. True.

180. False. Somatic passivity is a delusion.

181. True.

182. True. Can recognise an object and describe its functions, but cannot name them.

183. False. Speech and writing are affected though understanding is preserved.

184. True.

185. True.

186. False. Seen in Canadian Indians. It is the fear of engaging in cannibalism.

187. False. This is transsexualism.

188. False.

189. False. Free floating anxiety.

190. False. It is a screening test.

191. True.

Paper 4
Answers

192. True.

193. True.

194. False. Diffuse and less localised.

195. False. This is a positive symptom. The negative symptoms are muteness, withdrawal, apathy and anergia.

196. True.

197. True.

198. False. Form is the same though content varies.

199. False. Memory loss is generalised.

200. False.